The Healing Power *of*
TURMERIC

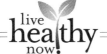

Warren Jefferson

live
hea|thy
now!

HEALTHY LIVING PUBLICATIONS
Summertown, Tennessee

© 2015 Warren Jefferson

Cover and interior design: Scattaregia Design

Healthy Living Publications,
a division of Book Publishing Company
PO Box 99
Summertown, TN 38483
888-260-8458
bookpubco.com

ISBN: 978-1-57067-324-5

Printed in the United States of America

20 19 18 17   2 3 4 5 6 7 8 9

Library of Congress Cataloging-in-Publication Data

Jefferson, Warren, 1943-
The healing power of turmeric / Warren Jefferson.
    pages cm
Includes bibliographical references.
ISBN 978-1-57067-324-5 (pbk.) -- ISBN 978-1-57067-863-9 (e-book)
1. Turmeric--Therapeutic use. I. Title.
RS165.T8J44 2015
615.3'2439--dc23
                    2015011992

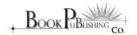

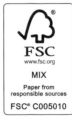

We chose to print this title on responsibly harvested paper stock certified by The Forest Stewardship Council,® an independent auditor of responsible forestry practices. For more information, visit us.fsc.org.org.

CONTENTS

Introduction

Despite the concerted efforts of conventional medical practitioners and scientific researchers to understand and effectively deal with both acute and chronic diseases, little has changed in well over fifty years in terms of how most common ailments are assessed and treated. Chronic diseases, such as cardiovascular and neurodegenerative conditions, diabetes, cancers, respiratory illnesses, and stroke comprise 46 percent of the total global disease burden and account for 59 percent of deaths worldwide. And these numbers aren't decreasing; alarmingly, they're on an upswing.

Current research has confirmed what traditional herbal healers have known for centuries: certain plants and plant-derived components can play valuable roles in critical healing processes, such as reducing inflammation, treating and preventing degenerative diseases, and even thwarting cancer. As a bonus, these plant-derived compounds are inexpensive, readily available, nontoxic, and devoid of the rampant and dangerous side effects that abound with the majority of pharmaceuticals.

These intriguing findings have piqued the interest of conventional as well as natural and alternative health care practitioners in nutraceuticals, which are food components that provide medicinal benefits encompassing the prevention and treatment of diseases. One of the most widely lauded natural plant components is curcumin, a pharmacologically active compound extracted from the rhizomes (tuber-shaped rootstalks) of the turmeric plant (*Curcuma longa*), a pungent, spicy-sweet herb.

Turmeric has been used medicinally for thousands of years. Initially it was used to help heal wounds, but it was also used to treat diverse conditions in traditional Ayurvedic and Asian medicine. More recently it has been discovered to also be capable of inhibiting the proliferation of cancer cells and blocking the pathways that induce chronic inflammation.

Turmeric, a plant related to ginger, is cultivated in India and other parts of Asia, and Africa, where it's widely used as a seasoning and regularly consumed in foods and beverages on a daily basis. Curcumin, the constituent in turmeric that's responsible for its naturally vibrant yellow color, is what gives curry powder its vivid hue. Known for its warm, bitter taste and golden color, turmeric is commonly added to Asian, African, and Indian seasonings, such as curry powders, and is used as a colorant in mustards, butter, and cheeses.

Turmeric has long been used in traditional Chinese medicine and Ayurvedic medicine as a treatment for inflammatory conditions, such as arthritis, colitis, and hepatitis. Its potent anti-inflammatory qualities present enormous therapeutic potential to combat a wide range of pro-inflammatory diseases, including but not limited to acute coronary syndrome, Alzheimer's disease, arthritis, atherosclerosis, cancers, cardiovascular disease, Crohn's disease, diabetes, gastric inflammation, gastric ulcer, pancreatitis, peptic ulcer, psoriasis, ulcerative colitis, ulcerative proctitis, uveitis (a form of eye inflammation), vitiligo, and others. The 2013 issue of *Current Pharmaceutical Design* reported that turmeric is effective in preventing and treating certain forms of cancer, including breast cancer. In addition, curcumin has been shown to be effective in treating alcohol intoxication, chronic arsenic exposure, hepatic conditions, and irritable bowel syndrome. It even shows promise as an antiaging agent!

Turmeric is used in cooking and in manufactured food products in many Western countries, and both turmeric and curcumin are available as dietary supplements. They both are listed as "generally regarded as safe" (GRAS) by the United States Food and Drug Administration (FDA). Human studies have shown curcumin to be safe at doses as high as 12 grams per day for three months. However, turmeric and curcumin are not currently approved as drugs, and more studies with human subjects are needed in order for curcumin to be approved to treat human disease.

The following pages explore what is currently known about turmeric and curcumin: their history, chemical and physical properties, and biological activity. In addition, you'll learn how turmeric has been a vital component of Ayurvedic and traditional Chinese medicine and read about its safety and recommended precautions for use. You'll also learn how to include turmeric in your diet and have a chance to try a few of my favorite recipes that include turmeric as a seasoning.

How a single natural biological agent can have so many health benefits has been a mystery to researchers for a long time. Fortunately, laboratory studies and clinical research have begun to give us a better understanding of curcumin and the potential of this amazing nutraceutical to treat and prevent a host of human diseases. Turmeric and curcumin might well be the long-awaited panacea that medical science has been searching for. So give turmeric a try. It's been proven safe to consume, and it just might make some great improvements in your health.

The History of Turmeric and Curcumin

Turmeric has a long history of use in many Asian cultures. At least four thousand years ago, the Vedic culture in India used it as a culinary spice, in religious ceremonies, and to treat a variety of medical conditions. Turmeric also has a long history of use in herbal remedies in the tropical regions of China and Indonesia.

Turmeric was introduced to Europe by Arab traders in the thirteenth century, but it wasn't until the late twentieth century that turmeric began to be used in the West as a dietary spice and therapeutic agent. In Ayurvedic and Asian folk medicine, turmeric is considered to have many medicinal properties and is used to treat a host of human ailments and conditions.

Curcumin is the most medicinally potent compound in turmeric. Although curcumin was known to have therapeutic effects as early as 1748, it was not until 1937 that curcumin was first tested on humans by a physician named Albert Oppenheimer, who at the time was an assistant professor of radiology at the American University of Beirut in Lebanon. He looked at curcumin's effect on human biliary disease, which is any illness that affects the gallbladder and its conduits. Oppenheimer found that an intravenous injection of a solution of 5 percent sodium curcumin resulted in the rapid emptying of the gallbladder. This was a significant medical breakthrough because increased bile flow activity could be beneficial in treating a variety of digestive disorders.

Oppenheimer went on to study curcumin's effect on inflammation of the gallbladder. In a study involving sixty-seven patients, he found that oral administration of curcumin completely cured the disease in all but one patient. In addition, there were no side effects reported, even though the medication was taken for many months.

In 1949 researchers published a paper in the scientific journal *Nature*, reporting that curcumin had antibacterial properties and was active against *Mycobacterium tuberculosis, Salmonella paratyphi, Staphylococcus aureus,* and *Trichophyton gypseum*. However, between 1940 and 1950, the American pharmaceutical industry transformed itself from a marginal collection of several hundred barely profitable firms to a small group of large, highly profitable corporations. It was likely due to this oligopoly and industry domination that natural medicinal remedies fell out of favor and scientists lost interest in curcumin. As a result, for the next twenty years there was not much research conducted on it.

Interest piqued again in the 1970s when three independent research groups discovered a number of new effects of curcumin, including its ability to lower cholesterol, reduce inflammation, regulate blood sugar levels in patients with diabetes, and increase antioxidant activity in the body. In 1980 an article published in the *Indian Journal of Medical Research* reported that curcumin had the potential to combat arthritis and was shown to have antirheumatic activity identical to phenylbutazone, a drug that at that time was commonly prescribed for arthritis. Curcumin was found to be well tolerated and didn't have any side effects. In 1987 a study published in the journal *Cancer Letters* showed that curcumin has anticancer activity and could effectively treat external cancerous lesions.

Since these initial results with curcumin, interest in the compound has increased appreciably. In the last twenty-five years, there have been over six thousand articles published in the National Institute of Health's PubMed database on the antioxidant, anti-inflammatory, antimicrobial, and anticancer activities of this amazing nutraceutical.

Biology of the Turmeric Plant

Turmeric is a product made from the tuberous roots (rhizomes) of the flowering perennial plant *Curcuma longa*, a member of the ginger family *Zingiberaceae*. It's a native of tropical South Asia and grows primarily in China, Haiti, Indonesia, India, Jamaica, the Philippines, and Taiwan. The plant has long oblong leaves and grows to a height of around three feet. *Curcuma longa* thrives in wet, hot climates between 68 and 86 degrees F.

The rhizomes of the turmeric plant contain the biologically active ingredients. Rhizomes are the underground stems of the plant; they grow horizontally, with small tubers branching off in all directions. They are yellow-brown with a dull orange interior and resemble gingerroot in overall appearance but are smaller. The main rhizome is typically three inches in length and one-half to one inch in diameter with a tapered end.

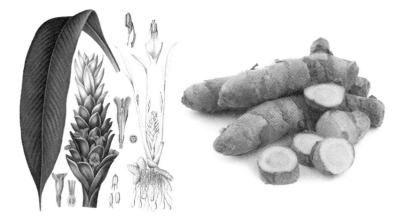

The plants are gathered annually for their rhizomes, and some are saved to reseed the following season. When the rhizome is dried, it's ground into a powder that has a yellow color and a slightly bitter, acetic yet sweet taste. This is what cooks the world over know as turmeric, an essential ingredient in curry powder and a seasoning that is widely used to flavor savory as well as sweet dishes.

Over one hundred thirty species of *Curcuma longa* have been identified worldwide, and the amount of curcumin they contain varies among the different species. India produces nearly all of the world's turmeric (500,000 metric tons) and exports about half of it. Indian turmeric is considered to be the best in the world because of its bright color and high curcumin content. The consumption of turmeric in Asian countries is reported to be in the range of 200 to 1,000 milligrams per day, or 160 to 440 grams per person per year!

Preparing Turmeric for Use

The turmeric rhizomes are boiled or steamed to remove some of the plant's odor and gelatinize the starch. This also produces a more uniform color to the finished product. Traditionally in India the rhizomes were boiled with cow dung, although this method is now discouraged for obvious health and sanitation reasons. In modern-day processing, the rhizomes are boiled in shallow pans in large iron pots containing alkalinized water, which is water containing a solution of sodium bicarbonate. The rhizomes are boiled for a minimum of forty minutes and as long as six hours, depending on the variety. The water is then drained and the rhizomes are dried in the sun until their moisture content reaches 8 to 10 percent. Next, the rhizomes are polished to remove the rough outer layer, and then they're ground into a powder.

Turmeric powder retains its color indefinitely, but the flavor could diminish over time. The powder is light sensitive, so it should be stored in an opaque container at room temperature to protect its potency.

Active and Nutritional Components of Turmeric

More than one hundred components have been isolated from the turmeric rhizomes. The main biologically active ones are the volatile essential oil of the plant containing turmerone, which is responsible for the aromatic qualities of turmeric, and three other agents called curcuminoids, which comprise between 2 and 9 percent of turmeric and produce its famous yellow coloring.

Curcumin, one of these curcuminoids, is practically insoluble in water but is soluble in acetone, dimethyl sulfoxide, ethanol, and methanol.

Curcumin is the principal curcuminoid, providing about 75 percent of the total curcuminoids in the plant. It is considered the most active constituent, showing potent pharmacological properties, including anticarcinogenic, anti-inflammatory, and antioxidant activity.

The dried rhizomes of turmeric contain on average between 3 and 6 percent curcumin. A standard-formula supplement of turmeric is supposed to contain 95 percent curcuminoids, but there's no guarantee of this because supplements are not totally regulated by the US Food and Drug Administration. Be sure to purchase your turmeric supplements from a manufacturer you are familiar with and have confidence in.

Table 1. Nutritional content in 100 grams of turmeric

Nutrient	Amount
Ascorbic acid	50 mg
Calcium	0.2 g
Calories	390
Carbohydrates	69.9 g
Cholesterol	0 mg
Fat, saturated	3 g
Fat, total	10 g
Fiber	21 g
Iron	47.5 mg
Niacin	4.8 mg
Phosphorous	0.26 g
Potassium	2,500 mg
Protein	8 g
Riboflavin	0.19 mg
Sodium	10 mg
Sugars	3 g
Thiamine	0.9 mg

Bioavailability of Curcumin

Curcumin is not water soluble, and this makes it difficult for the body to use it. Curcumin is poorly absorbed from the gastrointestinal tract, and when it's ingested by mouth, not much enters the bloodstream, so it has little effect in the body. A large dose must be taken orally before even small amounts get into the blood.

To increase the amount of curcumin that gets into the blood, piperine, an extract of black pepper, is often used in conjunction with curcumin. A study published in the journal *Planta Medica* in 1998 looked at the bioavailability of curcumin in healthy human volunteers. It showed that a dose of 2 grams of curcumin alone was very low and could not be detected in the blood. But when 20 milligrams of piperine was administered along with the curcumin, there was a much greater level detected. In fact, the added piperine increased blood levels of curcumin by 2,000 percent! So eating foods seasoned with both turmeric and black pepper will greatly enhance the absorption rate of the curcumin in the turmeric.

Curcumin is soluble in fat, so another way to increase its absorption is to take it with a little oil or other fat. When turmeric is included in a curry dish, for example, the curcumin is readily absorbed because there is usually some fat in the curry sauce. An enjoyable and effective way to absorb curcumin is drinking a traditional Ayurveduc beverage called golden milk tea (see the recipe on page 43), which can be made with coconut milk to supply the necessary fat.

Manufacturers have started to make small modifications to curcumin that could improve its solubility in water, enhance absorption rates, slow metabolism, and increase concentrations of curcumin in blood. These modifications are currently being tested and hold great promise.

Targeted Diseases

Curcumin is a polyphenol, which is a biologically active substance found in certain medicinal plants. Over three thousand studies conducted over the past twenty-five years, including both human and animal subjects, have demonstrated that curcumin has potent pharmacological properties. Although more studies specifically with human subjects are needed in order to understand the effective therapeutic dosage, safety precautions, and mechanisms involved to treat diseases, the following table lists the diseases turmeric has been shown to target.

Table 2. Diseases targeted by curcumin

Autoimmune diseases	Eczema
	Inflammatory bowel disease
	Irritable bowel syndrome
	Multiple sclerosis
	Psoriasis
	Scleroderma
Cancer	Bladder
	Bone
	Brain
	Breast
	Colon
	Esophagus
	Kidney
	Leukemia
	Lung
	Neck
	Pancreas
	Prostate
	Skin
	Stomach

Cardiovascular diseases	Atherosclerosis
	Cardiomyopathy
	Myocardial infarction
	Stroke
Inflammatory diseases	Allergy
	Arthritis
	Asthma
	Colitis
	Gallstones
	Sinusitis
	Ulcer
Liver diseases	Alcohol-induced liver disease
	Cirrhosis
	Fibrosis
	Jaundice
Lung diseases	Bronchitis
	Cystic fibrosis
	Hyaline membrane disease
Metabolic diseases	Alzheimer's disease
	Depression
	Diabetes
	Epilepsy
	Hyperlipidemia
	Hypoglycemia
	Hypothyroidism
	Lewy body disease
	Neurological diseases
	Obesity
	Parkinson's disease

Others	Antispasmodic sprain
	Cataract
	Fanconi anemia
	Fatigue
	Fever
	Hematuria
	Hemorrhage
	Osteoporosis
	Scabies
	Septic shock
	Wound healing

Turmeric in Ayurveda and Traditional Chinese Medicine

For thousands of years throughout Asia, turmeric has been used to prevent and treat a host of diseases. In addition to the conditions listed previously, there are other conditions that have been successfully treated with Ayurveda and traditional Chinese medicine.

Functions of Turmeric in Ayurveda and Traditional Chinese Medicine

antibacterial	antiseptic
anti-inflammatory	expectorant

Conditions Treated with Turmeric in Ayurveda and Traditional Chinese Medicine

allergy	bronchial congestion
anorexia	circulatory problems
arthritis	clogged blood vessels
asthma	cough
bloating	digestive disorders

flatulence	runny nose
gallstones	sinusitis
gas	skin conditions
irritable bowel syndrome	sore throat
lethargy	sprains
liver disorders	swelling
menstrual irregularity	worms
respiratory conditions	wounds

Metaflammation and Curcumin

Metaflammation and Chronic Disease

Many chronic diseases and conditions, including depression, heart disease, many forms of cancer, obesity, type 2 diabetes, and even dementia, have been associated with chronic inflammation, which is referred to as metaflammation because of its link with the metabolic system. Unlike classical inflammation that can sometimes play a healing role in chronic disease, metaflammation seems to aggravate and perpetuate disease rather than resolve it. This type of inflammation is characterized by specific attributes:

- It is low-grade, without a strong immune system response.
- It is chronic.
- It affects the whole body.
- It isn't produced by any recognizable foreign substance or injury that would typically cause an immune reaction.
- It is associated with a reduced rather than increased metabolic rate, as happens with classical inflammation.

Chronic diseases are those that are long-lasting, recurrent, noncommunicable, and not associated with a microbial infection. In many developed countries, chronic diseases account for as much as 70 percent of the disease burden among the population. Numerous studies have made the correlation between our modern lifestyle, metaflammation, and chronic disease.

Lifestyle Factors Associated with Metaflammation

The following lifestyle factors have a strong correlation with metaflammation:

- age
- consumption of trans-fatty acids
- depression
- high-fat diet
- inactivity
- inhalation of particulate matter
- obesity
- poor nutrition
- sleep deprivation
- smoking
- stress and anxiety
- weight gain

The following lifestyle factors have a moderately strong correlation with metaflammation:

- air pollution
- diets heavy in fast foods and processed meats
- economic insecurity
- high fructose intake
- high glucose intake
- high ratio of omega-6 to omega-3 fatty acids
- low fiber intake
- poor nutrition

Evidence correlating the following lifestyle factors with metaflammation is limited:

- endocrine-disrupting chemicals
- excessive alcohol consumption
- excessive exercise
- low socioeconomic status

- secondhand smoke
- sick-building syndrome
- starvation
- sugar-sweetened drinks
- thermal discomfort

It has been known for some time that foods cooked at high temperatures, especially meat, poultry, fish, and eggs, can create by-products that are very damaging to human health. The technical names for two of these by-products are advanced glycation end products (AGEs) and advanced lipoxidation end products (ALEs). In the body, AGEs and ALEs are potent inducers of inflammation.

Additionally, pasteurizing milk and the production and storage of milk powder create high levels of these by-products. Many foods, such as ice cream, special nutritional solutions and drinks, and baby formulas, are based on milk powder and its derivatives, which are processed at high temperatures. Consuming these food products adds to the body's inflammatory burden. People suffering from chronic diseases and those who are critically ill have an increased degree of inflammation or metaflammation in their body.

It stands to reason that if we could eliminate or at least moderate these inducers of metaflammation, we could possibly reduce the effects of chronic disease. A number of these lifestyle factors can be positively influenced and reduced by individuals, but some cannot. They simply come with living in the modern world.

Anti-inflammatory Activity of Curcumin

Curcumin is a potent anti-inflammatory with the potential to reduce and control metaflammation. In animal studies, cell culture studies, and clinical studies, curcumin has been shown to inhibit a number of factors that are involved in the inflammatory response, including inhibiting the expression of a gene that is involved.

Arthritis

In a study from Italy involving fifty patients with osteoarthritis of the knee, half of the subjects followed standard medical treatment, including taking nonsteroidal anti-inflammatory drugs (NSAIDs). The other half followed standard medical treatment and took a curcumin-based formulation. Patients taking the curcumin formulation showed a 58 percent reduction in overall pain and stiffness and improvement in physical functioning compared to the group that didn't take curcumin. They also showed a sixteenfold decrease in a marker for inflammation. The patients taking the curcumin formulation also showed a 300 percent improvement in emotional well-being compared to the group not taking the supplement.

This study showed that osteoarthritis patients could decrease the amount of prescribed medications they take and also increase the medications' efficacy. This is good news for patients when you consider that some pharmaceutical drugs to treat osteoarthritis have serious side effects and some have even been removed from the market because of significant safety concerns. A study published in the August 2009 issue of the *Journal of Alternative and Complementary Medicine* showed that turmeric extract worked as well as a nonsteroidal anti-inflammatory drug in the treatment of osteoarthritis of the knee.

Another study on osteoarthritis conducted at Siriraj Hospital in Bangkok, Thailand, divided 107 people who had osteoarthritis of the knee into two groups. People in one group were given 2 grams of turmeric per day and people in the second group were given 800 milligrams of ibuprofen per day. The trial lasted six weeks and at least forty-five people in each group completed the trial. At the end of the study, people in both groups reported improvements in their condition and rated themselves moderately to highly satisfied.

A preliminary intervention trial reported in the *Indian Journal of Medical Research* compared curcumin with a nonsteroidal anti-inflammatory drug (NSAID) in eighteen rheumatoid arthritis patients. Improvement was shown in morning stiffness, walking time, and joint swelling after two weeks of curcumin supplementation of 1,200 milligrams per day comparable to NSAID therapy of 300 milligrams per day for two weeks. A controlled clinical trial (a study in which participants are chosen at random to receive one of several clinical interventions measured against participants who do not receive the clinical intervention) reported in the medical journal *Phytotherapy Research* in the year 2000 used both a placebo and curcumin on forty hernia patients. The study found that oral curcumin supplementation of 1,200 milligrams per day for five days was more effective than a placebo in reducing swelling, tenderness, and pain after surgery and worked as well as phenylbutazone (a nonsteroidal anti-inflammatory) therapy of 300 milligrams per day.

Alzheimer's Disease

Turmeric may offer protection from Alzheimer's disease, which begins as an inflammatory process in the brain. Elderly populations in India have the lowest rates of the disease in the world, and it's thought that this might be because they eat turmeric with almost every meal. In an animal model of Alzheimer's disease, an injection of curcumin was found to cross the blood-brain barrier (a blockade of cells separating the circulating blood from elements of the central nervous system) and decreased biomarkers of inflammation and oxidative damage, plaque in the brain, and memory deficits.

Aluminum has been implicated as a possible cause of several neurodegenerative disorders, such as Alzheimer's and Parkinson's diseases. In a study done at Jawaharlal Nehru University in India in which lab rats were administered aluminum in their drinking water, it was reported that curcumin treatment weakened the poisonous effect of the aluminum by crossing the blood-brain barrier and binding with the metal. Because of these promising findings in animal studies, clinical trials of oral curcumin supplementation in patients with early Alzheimer's disease have begun.

Multiple Sclerosis

Curcumin may be helpful in treating multiple sclerosis patients. Multiple sclerosis (MS) is a disease in which the body's immune system attacks the protective sheath that covers the nerves. In a study conducted at Vanderbilt University Medical Center on mice with an MS-like disease, researchers found that curcumin blocked the progression of the disease. A second group of mice with the MS-like disease that were not treated with curcumin developed severe symptoms of the disease. In India and China, where turmeric is frequently consumed in meals, MS is rare.

Ocular Diseases

Two uncontrolled studies (those in which all the participants are given a treatment and there is no comparison with a control group not getting the treatment) suggest that oral curcumin supplementation of 1,125 milligrams per day for twelve weeks or longer improved chronic anterior uveitis, an inflammation of the iris of the eye. More research is needed to confirm this.

Cataract, a condition in which the eye lens becomes increasingly opaque, is the leading cause of blindness worldwide. Three different studies have shown curcumin to have significant preventive effects against this condition.

Additional Protective Capabilities of Curcumin

Anticancer Activity

Cancer is among the leading causes of sickness and death worldwide. In 2012 there were approximately 14 million new cases of cancer as well as 8.2 million deaths from cancer. Cancer can begin in any part of the body, and it manifests with rapid and abnormal cell growth that can invade adjoining parts of the body and spread, or metastasize, to other organs. This spreading to other areas of the body is the major way cancer kills.

The exact cause of cancer development and progression is not yet well understood, but it's thought to result from exposure to carcinogens that produce alterations in metabolic pathways (a series of chemical reactions occurring within a cell), genetic damage, and irreversible mutations. Current cancer treatment based on synthetic drugs, chemotherapy, and radiotherapy is expensive and also alters the various mechanisms of the normal actions of genes.

Curcumin has been shown to be an effective catalyst in an advanced therapeutic approach called targeted molecular therapy, which uses tumor antibodies, gene therapy, and other agents to dial down or completely shut off target genes that are causing uncontrolled cell growth. A number of studies have suggested that curcumin can exert a controlling influence on the molecules involved in almost every stage of cancer development by regulating the factors involved in cancer progression.

Curcumin has been shown to kill cancer cells in the breast, lungs, mouth, and prostate, as well as destroy human melanoma, myeloma, leukemia, and neuroblastoma cells. Oral doses of curcumin have been found to inhibit the development of chemically induced colon, liver, oral, and stomach cancer in animals. Human studies for cancer prevention and treatment with curcumin are being conducted, but they are in the very early stages.

Colorectal cancer is the second leading cause of cancer deaths in the United States. Currently there is no effective treatment except early detection and removal of the affected section of the colon, with or without chemotherapy, so the development of new therapies is an important goal for clinicians. A study published in 2002 in the medical journal *Cancer Epidemiology, Biomarkers & Prevention* found that when mice that were bred with a gene similar to the one that causes the development of colorectal cancer in humans were administered oral curcumin, the development of colon polyps was inhibited.

Numerous other clinical trials have shown curcumin to have potential against colorectal cancer. Curcumin is well absorbed into intestinal tissue and therefore might reduce the number of colon and rectal cancers.

An uncontrolled clinical study reported in 2001 in the medical journal *Clinical Cancer Research* showed that 15 patients with advanced colorectal cancer who were unresponsive to conventional treatment had a 59 percent reduction in cancer activity with the administration of an oral dose of curcumin extract of 440 milligrams taken daily for twenty-nine days. In five of these patients the disease was stabilized over the two- to four-month study period.

Turmeric was shown to be an effective antimutagen (a mutagen is a substance that changes the genetic material of an organism) in a study of chronic cigarette smokers reported in the medical journal *Mutagenesis* in 1992. The trial was done with sixteen chronic smokers and six nonsmokers who served as controls. The cigarette smokers were given 1.5 grams of turmeric per day for thirty days. A significant amount of mutagens is excreted in the urine of cigarette smokers, and smokers are likely to develop lung cancer. Turmeric dramatically reduced the urinary excretion of mutagens in the cigarette smokers, while no changes in the urinary excretion of mutagens were observed in the control group. The results indicated that dietary turmeric could be an effective antimutagen in cigarette smokers and reduce the risk of lung cancer.

Pancreatic cancer is the fourth leading cause of cancer deaths around the world. It's an insidious disease and can quickly develop to an advanced stage without any early warning symptoms. A clinical trial of twenty-five patients with advanced pancreatic cancer showed that curcumin was safe and well tolerated. The patients were given 8 grams of curcumin per day orally. Three patients showed improvement in markers for the disease, and the study concluded that curcumin is well tolerated in all patients and showed biological activity against pancreatic cancer in some patients.

While these studies and others are promising, especially with respect to colorectal cancer, larger, randomized, controlled clinical trials are necessary to confirm curcumin's clinical efficacy against cancer.

Antidepressive Activity

Major depression is a debilitating disorder affecting a growing number of people throughout the world. It's predicted to be the second most prevalent human illness by the year 2020. There are various antidepressants prescribed to alleviate the symptoms, but about 30 percent of depressed patients do not respond to existing drug therapies and 70 percent fail to achieve remission. Additionally, antidepressant drugs are associated with a number of serious side effects and compliance can be a problem.

Curcumin has shown promise against major depression in a number of animal models. Although how it brings about relief is not fully understood, it's thought that curcumin inhibits a neurotransmitter enzyme (a chemical that facilitates the transmission of signals between neurons across the synapses) and modulates the release of serotonin (a neurotransmitter that helps to maintain mood balance; a deficit of this chemical leads to depression), and dopamine (a neurotransmitter that helps control the brain's reward and pleasure centers; a deficiency results in Parkinson's disease and is associated with addiction). Curcumin also seems to enhance neurogenesis, the growth and development of nervous tissue, in the frontal cortex and hippocampal regions of the brain. More clinical studies are needed to determine if curcumin can indeed help major depression in humans.

Antidiabetic Activity

Curcumin has been shown to be effective against diabetes in patients. A clinical study was reported in the medical journal *Drugs in R&D* in 2008 in which seventy-two patients with type-2 diabetes were randomly given over the course of eight weeks either 300 milligrams of curcumin twice a day, 10 milligrams of atorvastatin (a cholesterol-lowering drug) once a day, or a placebo. Of the seventy-two patients, sixty-seven completed the study. The group given curcumin showed significant improvement in biomarkers for the disease. In another clinical trial, type-2 diabetes patients taking curcumin showed lower risk for the formation of plaques in the arteries by a reduction in insulin resistance, triglycerides, uric acid, visceral fat, and total body fat.

Curcumin might be able to delay the development of type-2 diabetes in prediabetic people. In a randomized, double-blind, placebo-controlled clinical trial published in the medical journal *Diabetes Care* in 2012, 240 participants were randomly assigned to receive either 1.5 grams of curcumin per day or placebo capsules. After nine months of treatment, 16.4 percent of the people in the placebo group were diagnosed with type-2 diabetes but none were diagnosed with the disease in the curcumin-treated group. The authors of the study felt that curcumin may be beneficial in preventing diabetes in people who haven't yet developed the disease.

Antioxidant Activity

Studies have demonstrated curcumin's powerful antioxidant activity by its ability to lower oxidative stress (damage caused by free radicals) in lab animals. A human study suggests that oral curcumin supplementation of 3.6 grams per day for seven days might inhibit oxidative DNA damage in patients with colorectal cancer. In a study relating to the eye, turmeric was shown to have minimized oxidative stress affecting the eye lens, indicating it could prevent or delay the development of cataracts.

Skin Protective Activity

Studies have suggested that curcumin is effective against numerous skin diseases, such as dermatitis, psoriasis, scleroderma, and skin cancer. In breast cancer patients, oral curcumin given during radiotherapy has been shown to reduce the severity of dermatitis from radiation treatments. Oral curcumin inhibited skin tumor development in laboratory mice. Curcumin is helpful in scleroderma (an autoimmune disease that can damage the organs) and other organ pathologies. In laboratory mice it relieved psoriasis-like inflammation. Numerous reports suggest that curcumin speeds up wound healing, prevents scar formation, and can help muscle regeneration.

Antimicrobial Activity of Curcumin

Antibacterial Activity

Despite some progress in the development of antibacterial agents, there is still the need to find new ones because of the evolution of multidrug-resistant bacteria. There's special interest in turmeric because it has been demonstrated in vitro (test tubes) that it has antibacterial activity against a wide variety of bacteria, including those listed in table 3, below.

Table 3. Bacteria that curcumin has been shown to be effective against

Bacterium	Location and role
Aeromonas hydrophila	Found in all freshwater environments and brackish water; could have a role in gastroenteritis.
Bacillus cereus	An anaerobic, spore-forming bacteria that is widespread in nature and in foods, especially in the spore state; causes food poisoning.
Bacillus subtilis	FDA listed as generally recognized as safe (GRAS), this very common bacteria is found in soil, water, air, and decomposing plant material.
Edwardsiella tarda	An uncommon enteric bacterium that has been found generally in animal hosts and occasionally in human feces; can cause irritation of the digestive tract, commonly referred to as stomach or intestinal flu.
Streptococcus agalactiae	Part of the normal flora of human intestines; can cause infection to newborn babies.

Staphylococcus aureus	Part of the normal skin flora; can cause arthritis, boils, bone infection, "flesh-eating bacteria" infection, genital infection, impetigo, life-threatening sepsis (staph blood invasion), pimples, pneumonia, sinusitis, staph infections, styes, toxic shock syndrome, and urinary tract infections.
Vibrio alginolyticus	The leading cause of seafood-related bacterial gastroenteritis and infectious diarrhea.
Vibrio cholerae	Causes cholera, an acute, diarrheal illness that can result in severe dehydration and even death within a matter of hours.
Vibrio harveyi	A natural inhabitant of seawater and a pathogen found in marine animals; thought to be the cause of the "milky seas effect," the uniform blue glow that is emitted from seawater at night.
Vibrio parahaemolyticus and *Vibrio vulnificus*	Found in warm coastal waters, such as the Gulf of Mexico; can cause disease in people who eat contaminated seafood; can also enter the body via a wound that is exposed to warm seawater; can cause bloodstream infections that are fatal in about 50 percent of victims.

Helicobacter pylori bacterium is a serious and widespread infectious agent and the common cause of peptic ulcers. This bacterium can also cause gastric cancer. The traditional treatment for peptic ulcers is with proton pump inhibitors and antibiotics, but these drugs are associated with a number of adverse side effects, such as abdominal pain, constipation, diarrhea, headache, nausea, and rash. Additionally, long-term use of these medications can increase the risk of osteoporosis-related fractures of the hip, wrist, or spine. Consequently, there is keen interest in developing alternative therapies to treat this condition. In an in vitro study, an extract of turmeric inhibited the growth of *Helicobacter pylori* as well as other bacteria. But two human trials with *H. pylori*-positive patients showed mixed results, and the authors concluded that curcumin showed limited antibactericidal effect on *H. pylori*. More studies with larger groups of participants are necessary to confirm whether there is a potential for curcumin against *H. pylori*.

In a clinical trial from Thailand, twenty-five patients with peptic ulcers were given two capsules of 300 milligrams each of turmeric orally five times a day over a period of four weeks. After four weeks ulcers were absent in twelve patients; after eight weeks ulcers were absent in eighteen patients; and after twelve weeks ulcers were absent in nineteen patients.

Synergistic Antibacterial Activity

Curcumin demonstrated a synergistic effect (a result of two combined agents that is greater than the the results of either agent alone) in combination with some antibiotics, including ampicillin, norfloxacin, and oxacillin against the dangerous methicillin-resistant *Staphylococcus aureus* (MRSA) strain. Additionally, the manufacture of silver nanocomposite films (bandages) impregnated with curcumin showed strong antibacterial activity against *Escherichia coli* (commonly called *E. coli*), a cause of problematic bacterial infections in hospitals, and could prove to be an effective antibacterial material for skin infections and burn and wound dressings.

Antifungal Activity

Systemic fungal infections, such as invasive candidiasis (*Candida*), have become a serious medical problem in the United States, affecting over ninety thousand people with compromised immune systems. *Candida* species have developed resistance to antifungal drugs, so finding new anti-*Candida* agents is crucial. In one study, the anti-*Candida* activity of curcumin was demonstrated against thirty-eight different strains of *Candida*, including some strains resistant to fluconazole (the drug treatment of choice) and clinical isolates of *Candida albicans*, *Candida glabrata*, *Candida guilliermondii*, *Candida krusei*, and *Candida tropicalis*. Turmeric oil has been shown to be effective in treating twenty-nine strains of fungi, including ringworm, that infect the skin, nails, and hair.

Antiviral Activity

Curcumin has a wide range of antiviral activity against a number of different viral pathogens, including parainfluenza virus type 3 (PIV-3), feline infectious peritonitis virus (FIPV), vesicular stomatitis virus (VSV), herpes simplex virus (HSV), flock house virus (FHV), and respiratory syncytial virus (RSV). In test tube studies, curcumin showed anti-influenza activity against a number of influenza viruses, namely PR8, H1N1, and H6N1. Unlike amantadine, which is used to treat influenza, viruses developed no resistance to curcumin in these tests.

An in vitro study of curcumin showed strong antiviral activity against herpes simplex virus type 1 (HSV-1), and an in vivo study (a study done on living organisms) on mice with intravaginal herpes simplex virus type 2 (HSV-2), curcumin gave protection from infection. These tests showed that curcumin could be a good candidate for developing intravaginal products for protection against sexually transmitted herpes virus infections. Additionally, curcumin has shown to have potent antiviral effects against hepatitis B and hepatitis C viruses as well as adult T-cell leukemia in in vitro tests.

Available Forms and Dosage Recommendations

Turmeric is available in the following forms:

- Capsules containing powder
- Dried root
- Fluid extract
- Loose powder
- Raw root
- Tablets
- Tincture

Dried Root

Turmeric powder, made from the dried root, is the most common form of the herb. It's typically used as a culinary seasoning, mixed with juice or other beverages, or consumed in a capsule. The US National Institutes of Health have stated that adults in India consume on average between 2 and 2.5 grams (roughly .75 ounce) of dried turmeric root daily. The University of Maryland Medical center notes that between 1.5 and 3 grams per day is an appropriate dose for an average-sized adult. A health care provider may recommend a specific dose of turmeric depending on an individual's age, weight, and medical condition. Turmeric supplements haven't been studied in children, so there is no recommended dose. Do not administer to children and do not take if you are pregnant or breastfeeding.

Standardized Turmeric Powder

Some supplement manufacturers offer turmeric powder and other products that contain a guaranteed concentration of curcumin. The University of Maryland Medical Center recommends 400 to 600 milligrams of standardized turmeric powder three times day for an average-sized adult. Standardized turmeric powder hasn't been studied in children, so there is no recommended dose. Do not administer to children and do not take if you are pregnant or breastfeeding.

Turmeric Tea

The National Institutes of Health recommends steeping half an ounce of turmeric root in 4.5 ounces of boiling-hot water. This preparation may be taken twice daily. Do not administer to children and do not take if you are pregnant or breastfeeding.

Fluid Extract

The University of Maryland Medical Center recommends 30 to 90 drops per day of an aqueous (water-based) turmeric extract in one-to-one dilution. Extracts may provide medicinal benefits similar to the dried powder or tea. Do not administer to children and do not take if you are pregnant or breastfeeding.

Tincture

Tinctures made with alcohol may be used to create concentrated liquid turmeric supplements. The University of Maryland Medical Center recommends taking 15 to 30 drops four times daily for an average-sized adult. Because tinctures contain alcohol, they should not be given to children, women who are pregnant or breastfeeding, or people with liver disease.

Safety and Precautions

Although the use of herbs is a time-honored approach for improving health, treating disease, and strengthening the immune system, herbs should nevertheless be used with care and caution. Some herbs can trigger side effects and may negatively interact with other herbs, supplements, prescription drugs, or over-the-counter medications. When using turmeric or any other herb, always do so under the supervision of a qualified health care provider.

In cooking, turmeric is considered safe, the same as any other culinary herb or seasoning. That's because the amount ingested at a meal is typically small, even though when consumed over extended periods of time, turmeric used in recipes may have positive effects on health.

Turmeric and curcumin supplements haven't been tested on children and aren't recommended for use by them or by women who are pregnant or breastfeeding. When taken at the recommended dosages by all other adults, the supplements are considered safe. However, large amounts of turmeric supplements ingested over long periods of time might cause stomach upset and, in extreme cases, ulcers. People who have gallstones, liver disease, or obstruction of the bile passages should talk to their doctors before taking turmeric or curcumin.

Turmeric may lower blood sugar levels. While this is viewed as a positive effect by most people, individuals with diabetes should consult with their doctors before taking turmeric supplements. The combination of turmeric and diabetes medications could cause hypoglycemia (low blood sugar).

Turmeric has blood-thinning capacities. Stop taking turmeric supplements at least two weeks prior to having surgery, and be sure to tell your doctor and surgeon that you've been taking turmeric.

If you are being treated with any of the medications listed in table 4, below, avoid taking turmeric or curcumin supplements without first getting clearance from your health care provider.

Table 4. Drugs with which turmeric supplements might interact

Type of mediation	Name
Antacids	Alka-Seltzer
	Gelusil
	Maalox
	Mylanta
	Pepto-Bismol
	Rolaids
	Tums

Blood thinners	Apixaban (Eliquis)
	Aspirin
	Clopidogrel bisulfate (Plavix)
	Dabigatran (Pradaxa)
	Ibuprofen (Advil, Nuprin, Motrin)
	Naproxen sodium (Aleve, Aflaxen, Anaprox)
	Rivaroxaban (Xarelto)
	Warfarin (Coumadin, Jantoven, Marevan, Uniwarfin)
Diabetes medications	Alpha-glucosidase inhibitors
	Biguanides
	Bile acid sequestrants
	DPP-4 inhibitors
	Meglitinides
	SGLT2 inhibitors
	Sulfonylureas
	Thiazolidinediones
H_2 blockers	Cimetidine (Tagamet)
	Famotidine (Calmicid, Fluxid, Pepcid)
	Nizatidine (Axid)
	Ranitidine (Tritec, Zantac)
Protein pump inhibitors (PPIs)	Esomeprazole (Nexium)
	Lansoprazole (Prevacid)
	Omeprazole (Prilosec, Zegerid)
	Pantoprazole (Protonix)
	Rabeprazole (Aciphex)

Conclusion

Phytochemical analysis of turmeric has shown that this amazing nutraceutical contains a large number of biologically active compounds, including curcumin, curcuminoids, and volatile oil. In numerous in vitro, in vivo, and human clinical studies, curcumin, the most biologically active compound in turmeric, has been shown to have potent pharmacological properties. It's able to interact with multiple molecular targets and has therapeutic value and potential against a wide array of human diseases. Curcumin has been found to be active against bacteria, inflammation, oxidants, tumors, and viruses. In addition, it is an antiseptic; protects the heart, liver, kidneys, and digestive system; and reduces damage cause by radiation. Clinical human studies have confirmed the safety, tolerability, and nontoxicity of curcumin even at high doses of up to 12 grams per day.

The beneficial effects of turmeric have traditionally been acquired from eating foods seasoned with the herb over a long period of time, such as in India, where people eat turmeric at almost every meal. Today people in the West can get the benefits of this healthful herb by taking turmeric or curcumin dietary supplements, available in most natural food stores.

There's been a lot of research on curcumin over the past twenty-five years, and scientists have learned a great deal about it, but there are still many unanswered questions. It is hoped that ongoing and future laboratory studies and human clinical trials with turmeric and curcumin will lead to an increased understanding of the full therapeutic potential of this amazing plant.

Recipes

Curried Potatoes with Cauliflower

Makes 4 servings

This traditional Indian dish, known as *aloo gobi*, is surprisingly quick and easy to make yet is incredibly rich in flavor. The turmeric imparts an eye-appealing golden color.

2 tablespoons whole garlic cloves

2 tablespoons peeled and sliced fresh ginger

1 tablespoon olive oil

1 tablespoon ground coriander

½ teaspoon ground turmeric

1 cup water

2 tablespoons peanut oil

1 large serrano chile, split in half lengthwise

1 teaspoon whole cumin seeds

1 small head cauliflower, cut into small florets

2 russet potatoes, peeled and cubed

Salt

2 tablespoons minced fresh cilantro or parsley, for garnish

Put the garlic, ginger, and olive oil in a food processor and pulse into a fairly smooth paste. Measure out 2 tablespoons of the paste and put it in a small bowl. Store the rest of the paste in a covered container in the refrigerator for another use. Add the coriander, turmeric, and ½ cup of the water to the garlic paste and stir to combine.

Put the peanut oil in a large saucepan over medium-high heat. When the oil is hot, add the chile, wait 30 seconds, and then add the cumin. Stir in the garlic mixture and cook, stirring frequently, for 2 minutes.

Add the cauliflower and potatoes and stir until evenly coated with the seasonings. Add the remaining ½ cup of water, cover, and cook over medium heat, stirring occasionally, for 15 minutes. Uncover and cook, stirring occasionally, until the cauliflower and potatoes are tender, about 5 minutes longer. Season with salt to taste. Serve hot, garnished with the cilantro.

Curried Ginger-Squash Soup

Makes 4 servings

This satisfying soup, made with just the right amount of spice, is warming and welcoming, especially in chilly weather.

3 cups water

1 small pumpkin, or 1 medium butternut squash, unpeeled and cut into 2-inch chunks

1 cup chopped leek or red onion

1 apple, diced (peeling optional)

3 cloves garlic, minced

1 (2-inch) piece fresh ginger, peeled and minced

1 teaspoon green curry paste, or 1 small jalapeño chile, minced

2 tablespoons maple syrup

2 tablespoons olive oil

2 tablespoons tamari

1 teaspoon ground cinnamon

1 teaspoon ground turmeric

1 teaspoon ground coriander

½ teaspoon whole cumin seeds

½ teaspoon ground pepper

½ teaspoon salt

Put the water in a large soup pot. Put a steamer basket in the pot and bring the water to a boil over high heat. Put the pumpkin in the steamer basket, cover, and steam until fork-tender, about 15 minutes. Transfer the pumpkin to a colander and remove the steamer basket from the pot but do not drain the pot.

Put the leek, apple, garlic, ginger, and curry paste in the pot with the hot water. Cover and remove from the heat.

Rinse the pumpkin under cold water until it is cool enough to handle. Remove and discard the peel. Put the pumpkin flesh, the leek mixture, and the maple syrup, oil, tamari, cinnamon, turmeric, coriander, cumin, pepper, and salt in a blender (you might have to do this in batches depending on the size of your blender) and process until smooth. Return to the soup pot and heat over medium heat until steaming hot.

Recipe from *The Ayurvedic Vegan Kitchen* by Talya Lutzker.

Mom's Mac and Cheese

Makes 8 servings

There's nothing quite as comforting as macaroni and cheese, whether you're feeling down in the dumps or want to celebrate. Here's a delicious dairy-free version of this nourishing classic.

4 cups whole-grain elbow macaroni

3 tablespoons plus 2 teaspoons coconut oil

3 cups unsweetened almond milk

2 tablespoons stone-ground mustard

1 tablespoon dried rosemary

2 teaspoons whole cumin seeds

2 teaspoons dried basil

1 teaspoon salt

1 teaspoon ground coriander

1 teaspoon ground turmeric

1 cup shredded vegan Cheddar cheese

¼ cup chopped fresh basil or parsley, for garnish

Cook the macaroni in boiling water in a large saucepan according to the package directions. Drain, rinse, and return to the saucepan. Add 1 teaspoon of the oil and stir until evenly distributed.

Preheat the oven to 375 degrees F. Lightly oil a 13 x 9-inch glass baking dish with 1 teaspoon of the oil.

Put the almond milk in a medium saucepan and warm over medium-high heat for 1 minute. Add the remaining 3 tablespoons of oil and the mustard, rosemary, cumin, dried basil, salt, coriander, and turmeric. Stir until the coconut oil is melted and the seasonings are evenly distributed. Remove from the heat and stir in the cheese. Pour the sauce over the macaroni and stir until well combined. Pour the macaroni mixture into the prepared baking dish. Bake for 35 minutes. Increase the heat to 425 degrees F and bake for 10 minutes longer, or until the top is golden brown. Garnish with the fresh basil just before serving.

Recipe from *The Ayurvedic Vegan Kitchen* by Talya Lutzker.

Okra Curry

Makes 6 servings

Okra originated in Africa but is used extensively in the Middle East, India, and Sri Lanka. In the United States, okra most often appears in the gumbo soups featured in Creole cuisine. Young okra is preferred for this recipe. With only a quick fry, it will retain its crunchy texture. But if you prefer it softer, you can cook it slowly in the sauce to bring out its characteristically gummy texture.

Seasoned Okra

1 pound young okra, trimmed and thinly sliced crosswise

1 teaspoon ground turmeric

1 teaspoon ground dried chiles or paprika

½ teaspoon salt

½ cup vegetable oil

Curry Sauce

1 cup chopped yellow onion

3 tablespoons minced green jalapeño or serrano chiles

2 teaspoons ground coriander

1 teaspoon ground cumin

1 cinnamon stick

6 fresh or dried curry leaves or bay leaves

1 teaspoon salt

1 cup full-fat coconut milk

To make the seasoned okra, put the okra, turmeric, ground chiles, and salt in a mixing bowl. Toss until the seasonings are evenly distributed.

Heat the oil in a medium saucepan or wok over medium heat. Add the okra in small batches and fry until cooked but still crunchy, 2 to 3 minutes. Drain on absorbent paper.

To make the sauce, add the onion to the remaining oil in the pan and cook over medium heat, stirring frequently, until light brown and fragrant, 2 to 3 minutes. Add the chiles, coriander, cumin, cinnamon stick, curry leaves, and salt. Stir in the coconut milk, decrease the heat to low, and simmer for 10 minutes, stirring occasionally.

For crispy okra, serve the sauce on the side. For soft okra, add the okra to the pan with the sauce and toss until evenly coated. Serve immediately.

Recipe from *Asian Fusion* by Chat Minkwan.

Lentil and Spinach Dal

Makes 6 servings

Dal refers to Indian lentils or the dishes that are made with them. This version of dal has spinach added. Assorted spices are essential for obtaining the complex, aromatic flavors. As dried beans take a while to cook and fresh spinach cooks very quickly, make sure that the lentils have just the right texture before adding the spinach for the final touch.

¼ cup vegetable oil

2 teaspoons brown mustard seeds

2 green jalapeño or serrano chiles, cut lengthwise into quarters

¼ cup peeled and minced fresh ginger

1½ cups yellow split lentils or peas, or split chana dal, rinsed well and drained

6 cups vegetable broth or water

1 vegetable bouillon cube

1 tablespoon sugar

2 teaspoons ground cumin

2 teaspoons ground coriander

1 teaspoon ground turmeric

½ teaspoon asafetida or garlic powder

½ teaspoon salt

1 pound fresh spinach leaves, stemmed

1 cup thinly sliced green onions

Heat the oil in a large soup pot over medium heat. Stir in the mustard seeds, chiles, and ginger. Cook, stirring occasionally, until the mustard seeds start to jump and crackle and the chiles sizzle, 2 to 3 minutes. Transfer to a small bowl and set aside.

Put the lentils and vegetable broth in the same pot used for the mustard seeds and bring to a boil over high heat. Decrease the heat to low and cook, stirring occasionally, for 8 to 10 minutes, skimming off any foam that rises to the surface.

Stir in the bouillon cube, sugar, cumin, coriander, turmeric, asafetida, and salt. Partially cover the pot with a lid and simmer, stirring occasionally, until the lentils are very tender and only a little liquid is left on top, 35 to 40 minutes.

Stir in the spinach and green onions. Cook, stirring frequently, until the spinach is wilted, 4 to 6 minutes. If the mixture seems dry, add a little water to achieve the desired consistency.

Transfer to a serving platter. Sprinkle with the reserved mustard seed mixture.

Recipe from *Asian Fusion* by Chat Minkwan.

Potato Subji

Makes 7 servings

India's vegetarian tradition has roots in antiquity, and Indian cooking has a great deal to offer in terms of color, depth, richness, and variety. For example, this vegetable dish (*subji*) is one of the tastiest potato recipes imaginable.

2 tablespoons coconut oil or extra-virgin olive oil

1 tablespoon brown mustard seeds

2 cups diced onions

2 teaspoons ground turmeric

4 russet, gold, or red-skinned potatoes, scrubbed and cubed

¼ cup water, plus more if needed

1 teaspoon salt

Put the oil and mustard seeds in a large saucepan over medium heat. After the seeds begin to pop, cover, and cook until you hear that the seeds have stopped popping, 1 to 2 minutes.

Stir in the onions and cook, stirring frequently, until soft, 3 to 5 minutes. Stir in the turmeric and cook, stirring occasionally, for 1 minute. Stir in the potatoes, water, and salt. Cover and cook, stirring occasionally, until the potatoes are fork-tender, about 20 minutes. Add a little more water during cooking if necessary to keep the potatoes from drying out.

Recipe from *Cooking Vegan* by Vesanto Melina and Joseph Forest.

Southwest Scrambled Tofu

Makes 6 servings

Ground turmeric gives this dish a golden hue reminiscent of eggs.

1 pound medium or firm tofu, drained and crumbled

1 tablespoon tamari

1 tablespoon vegetable oil

1 small red or green bell pepper, diced

1 cup sliced mushrooms

½ cup sliced green onions

1 small tomato, chopped

2 tablespoons nutritional yeast flakes

1 teaspoon ground turmeric

2 cloves garlic, minced

½ teaspoon hot sauce

2 tablespoons chopped fresh cilantro or parsley

Salt

Ground black pepper

Salsa (optional)

Crumble the tofu into a medium bowl. Add the tamari and mix until evenly distributed.

Heat the oil in a large skillet over medium heat. Add the bell pepper, mushrooms, and green onions. Cook, stirring occasionally, for 4 minutes. Add the tofu and tomato and stir to combine. Add the nutritional yeast, turmeric, garlic, and hot sauce and stir to combine. Cover and cook, stirring occasionally, for 10 minutes. If the mixture seems dry, add 1 to 2 teaspoons of water as needed. Add the cilantro and stir until evenly distributed. Season with salt and pepper to taste. Serve with a dollop of salsa on top or on the side if desired.

Turmeric Tea

Makes 4 servings

This is an enjoyable way to get more turmeric into your diet. The tea is both warming and soothing.

4 cups water

1 teaspoon grated fresh turmeric or ground turmeric

1 teaspoon grated fresh ginger or ground ginger (optional)

Sweetener (optional)

Lemon juice (optional)

Put the water in a medium saucepan and bring to a boil over high heat. Add the turmeric and optional ginger, decrease the heat to medium, and simmer, stirring occasionally, for 10 minutes. Strain through a fine-mesh sieve into a teacup or mug. Add sweetener and lemon juice to taste if desired.

Golden Coconut Milk Tea

Makes 2 servings

It's hard to believe that a beverage this delicious is also quite healthy. Enjoy it with breakfast, as a snack or treat, or as an after-dinner drink instead of coffee. The black pepper will help your body better absorb the curcumin in the turmeric.

    1 can (8 ounces) full-fat coconut milk
    1 cup water
    1 teaspoon ground turmeric
    1 teaspoon ground cinnamon
    1 teaspoon maple syrup
    Pinch black pepper

Put all the ingredients in a blender and process until smooth. Pour into a small saucepan and heat over medium heat, stirring occasionally, until hot but not boiling, 3 to 5 minutes. Serve immediately.

Video Resources

 Curcumin A Big Medicine—
Turmeric Curcumin
Health Talk
youtu.be/01PcxCgtgr4

 Curcumin Reduces Risk of
HPV-Related
Cervical Cancer
youtu.be/2yJoE7F2lM8

 Curcumin and Your Health
youtu.be/SWbHFIb6r6Q

 How Curcumin Helps
Prevent and Treat Cancer
youtu.be/QNLt1fZR1Bl

 Cancer Cure | Turmeric |
Natural Cancer Cure
youtu.be/jqj6EqjSWW8

 Smart Tips—Anti-Cancer
Kitchen Spice
youtu.be/tvahuahhrZw

 Curcumin for colon cancer
youtu.be/elQFAv6hNRo

 The Benefits of Curcumin
youtu.be/ZHu280-mf7E

 Curcumin for the Prevention
of Polyps for FAP (familial
adenomatous polyposis)
youtu.be/e7EGeVTBbqw

 Theracurmin—A Major
Breakthrough
in Curcumin Absorption
youtu.be/EQYnkOkc6C8

 Curcumin Kills Cancer Cells
youtu.be/pAzwGKC_Cls

 Turmeric: Naturally Reverse
Cancer, Arthritis, and
Inflammation
youtu.be/YS-nyqBJeGc

 Curcumin May Help Prevent
Type 2 Diabetes
youtu.be/KnAW-aQZk6U

References

Bengmark, S., and G. Mesa. 2009. "Plant-Derived Health: The Effects of Turmeric and Curcuminoids." *Nutr Hisp* 281-473.

Bundy, R., and A. Walker et al. 2004. "Turmeric Extract May Improve Irritable Bowel Syndrome Symptomatology in Otherwise Healthy Adults: A Pilot Study." *The Journal of Alternative and Complementary Medicine* 10 (6): 1015–1018.

Clement, B. 2013. *Food Is Medicine: Volume Two*. Summertown, TN: Hippocrates Publications.

Davis, B., and V. Melina. 2013. *Becoming Vegan: Express Edition*. Summertown, TN: Book Publishing Company.

Egger, G. 2012. "In Search of a Germ Theory Equivalent for Chronic Disease." *Prev Chronic Dis* 9:110301. doi:10.5888/pcd9.110301.

Garcea, G., D. Jones, and R. Singh et al. 2004. "Detection of Curcumin and Its Metabolites in Hepatic Tissue and Portal Blood of Patients Following Oral Administration." *Br J Cancer* 90 (5):1011–1015.

Gupta, S., and S. Patchca et al. 2015. "Therapeutic Roles of Curcumin: Lessons Learned from Clinical Trials." *The AAPS Journal* 15 (1):195–218. doi:10.1208/s12248-012-9432-8.

Kulkarni, S. K. et al. 2009. "Potentials of Curcumin as an Antidepressant." *The Scientific World Journal* 9:1233–1241. doi:10.1100/tsw.2009.137.

Kuttan, R., P. Bhanumathy, K. Nirmala, and M. George. 1985. "Potential Anticancer Activity of Turmeric (*Curcuma longa*)." *Cancer Lett* 29:197–202.

Lee, W. H. et al. 2013. "Curcumin and Its Derivatives: Their Application in Neuropharmacology and Neuroscience in the 21st Century." *Current Neuropharmacology* 11:338–378. ncbi.nlm.nih.gov/pmc/articles/PMC3744901/pdf/CN-11-338.pdf.

Linus Pauling Institute. "Curcumin." lpi.oregonstate.edu/infocenter/phytochemicals/curcumin.

Moghadamtousi, S. et al. 2014. "A Review on Antibacterial, Antiviral, and Antifungal Activity of Curcumin." *BioMed Research International*. doi:10.1155/2014/186864.

Oppenheimer, A. 1937. "Turmeric (Curcumin) in Biliary Diseases." *The Lancet* 229 (5924):619-621.

Perkins, S., R. Verschoyle, and K. Hill et al. 2002. "Chemopreventive Efficacy and Pharmacokinetics of Curcumin in the Min/+ Mouse, a Model of Familial Adenomatous Polyposis." *Cancer Epidemiol Biomarkers Prev* 11 (6):535–540.

Polasa, K., T. Raghuram, and T. Krishna et al. 1992. "Effect of Turmeric on Urinary Mutagens in Smokers." *Mutagenesis* 7 (2):107.

Prasad, S., and B. Aggarwal. 2011. "Turmeric, the Golden Spice: From Traditional Medicine to Modern Medicine." In *Herbal Medicine: Biomolecular and Clinical Aspects,* edited by I. Benzie and S. Wachtel-Galor. Boca Raton, FL: CRC Press.

Prasad, S., and S. Gupta et al. 1994. "Curcumin, a Component of Golden Spice: From Bedside to Bench and Back." *Biotechnology Advances* 32 (6): 1053–1064. ncbi.nlm. nih.gov/books/NBK92752.

Rahmani, A. et al. 2014. "Curcumin: A Potential Candidate in Prevention of Cancer via Modulation of Molecular Pathways." *BioMed Research International.* doi:10.1155/2014/761608.

Schraufstatter, E., and H. Bernt. 1949. "Antibacterial Action of Curcumin and Related Compounds." *Nature* 164:456.

Sethi, P. et al. 2009. "Curcumin Attenuates Aluminum-Induced Functional Neurotoxicity in Rats." *Pharmacol Biochem Behav* 93 (1): 31–9. doi:10.1016/j. pbb.2009.04.005.

Sharma, R. et al. 2001. "Pharmacodynamic and Pharmacokinetic Study of Oral Curcuma Extract in Patients with Colorectal Cancer." *Clinical Cancer Research* 7 (7):1894–1900.

Shishodia, S. et al. 2005. "Curcumin: Getting Back to the Roots." *Annals of the New York Academy of Sciences* 1056:206–217. doi:10.1196/annals.1352.010.

University of Maryland Medical Center. "Turmeric." umm.edu/health/medical/ altmed/herb/turmeric.

Uribarri, J. et al. 2010. "Advanced Glycation End Products of Foods and a Practical Guide to Their Reduction in the Diet." *J Am Diet Assoc* 110 (6):911–16.e12. doi:10.1016/j.jada.2010.03.018.

Weil, A. 2015. "Turmeric Health Benefits: Have a Happy New Year with Turmeric." *Huffington Post.* huffingtonpost.com/andrew-weil-md/turmeric-health-have-a-happy-new-year_b_798328.html.

Weil, A. 2003. "Turmeric for MS." drweil.com/drw/u/id/QAA288736.

WHO (World Health Organization). 2015. "Fact Sheet No. 297: Cancer." who.int/ mediacentre/factsheets/fs297/en.

About the Author

Warren Jefferson is a research writer for Book Publishing Company. He's the author of four other health titles: *Colloidal Silver Today, The Neti Pot for Better Health, Understanding Gout,* and *Enhance Your Health with Fermented Foods.*

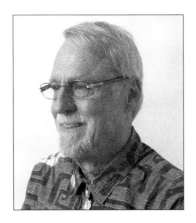

Also by Warren Jefferson:

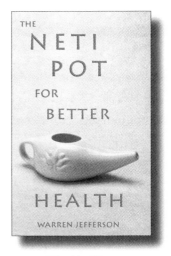

The Neti Pot
for Better Health
978-1-57067-186-9
$9.95

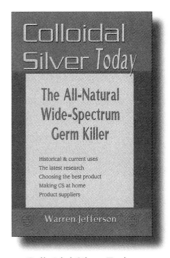

Colloidal Silver Today
978-1-57067-154-8
$6.95

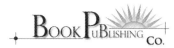

BOOK PUBLISHING CO.

books that educate, inspire, and empower

All titles in the **Live Healthy Now** series are only **$5.95!**

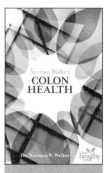

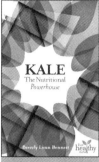

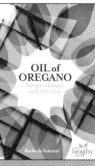

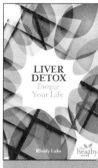

HEALTH ISSUES	HEALTHY FOODS	HERBS AND SUPPLEMENTS	NATURAL SOLUTIONS
SUGAR DETOX Defeat Cravings and Restore Your Health	Enhance Your Health with **FERMENTED FOODS**	**OLIVE LEAF EXTRACT** The Mediterranean Healing Herb	The Healing Power of **TURMERIC**
THE ACID-ALKALINE DIET Balancing the Body Naturally	**GREEN SMOOTHIES** The Easy Way to Get Your Greens	**AROMATHERAPY** Essential Oils for Healing	Weight Loss and Good Health with **APPLE CIDER VINEGAR**
GLUTEN-FREE Success Strategies	**PALEO** Smoothies	The Pure Power of **MACA**	Healthy and Beautiful with **COCONUT OIL**
A Holistic Approach to **ADHD**	Refreshing Fruit and Vegetable **SMOOTHIES**		The Weekend **DETOX**
Understanding **GOUT**			Improve Digestion with **FOOD COMBINING**
WHEAT BELLY Is Modern Wheat Causing Modern Ills?			

See our complete line of titles at **BookPubCo.com** or order directly from:
Book Publishing Company • PO Box 99 • Summertown, TN 38483 • 1-888-260-8458
Free shipping on all book orders